I0765273

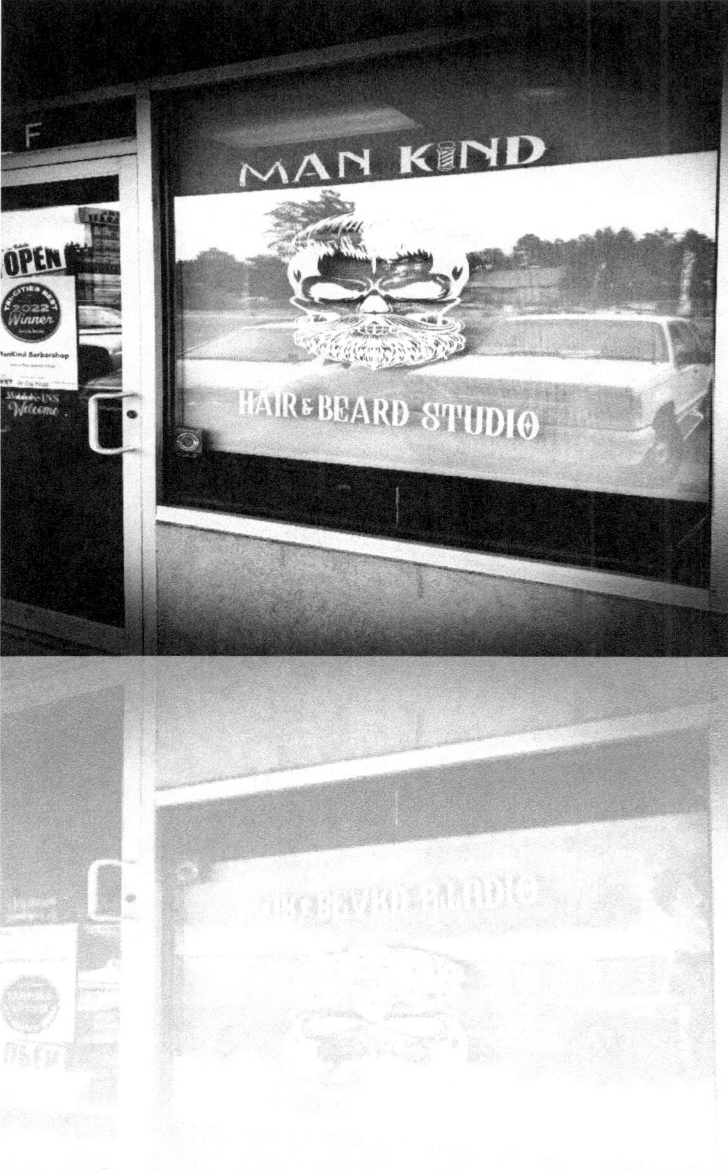
F
OPEN
2022
Winner
ManKind Barbershop
WALK-INS
Welcome
MAN KIND
HAIR & BEARD STUDIO

All rights reserved.

No part of this publication may be reproduced, stored in a retrieval system, or transmitted, in any form or by any means, electronic, mechanical, photocopying, recording or otherwise, without the prior written permission of the presenters.

Heather Mortensen asserts the moral right to be identified as author of this work.

Chapter 1: The Journey Begins: How I Became a Men's Hairstylist

Early Passion for Hair: My Childhood Fascination

From a young age, I was captivated by the world of hair. While other kids were playing with trucks and dolls, I found myself mesmerized by the artistry and creativity that went into styling hair. This early passion for hair sparked a journey that would eventually lead me to become a men's hairstylist, specializing in the art of beard grooming. In this subchapter, I want to take you back to my childhood and share the story of how my fascination with hair began.

Growing up, I was always drawn to the salon in my grandmother's basement. Later, a friend s mother's home salon. the smell of perms and the camaraderie among patrons created an atmosphere that was both exciting and comforting. I would sit for hours, observing the barbers' skilled hands as they transformed unkempt hair into works of art.

It was in a barbershop that I discovered my true calling.

As I entered my teenage years, my passion for hair actually disappeared and it wasn't until I was a newly divorced mom of two toddlers that I considered a career in it

After completing my formal training as a hairstylist, I found myself gravitating towards the world of men's grooming. There was something about the art of beard styling that intrigued me like no other. The ability to transform a rugged beard into a polished and well-groomed masterpiece became my ultimate goal.

Becoming a men's hairstylist allowed me to combine my childhood fascination with my passion for beard grooming. I honed my skills, attending seminars and workshops to stay up-to-date with the latest trends and techniques. Over the years, I have had the privilege to work with countless clients, each with their unique beard aspirations and desires.

In this book, "Confessions of a Men's Hairstylist: Insider Tips for Beard Enthusiasts," I aim to share my wealth of knowledge and experiences with potential beard clients like yourself. Whether you are looking for tips on beard maintenance, styling, or choosing the right grooming products, this book will guide you every step of the way.

Join me on this journey as we delve into the world of men's grooming, where passion and creativity merge to create the perfect beard. Together, we will unlock the secrets to achieving the beard of your dreams, while exploring the artistry and satisfaction that comes with being a men's hairstylist. It's time to embrace your inner beard enthusiast and embark on a transformative grooming adventure.

Discovering My Talent: First Steps in Hairstyling

For all the potential beard clients out there who have ever considered diving into the world of hairstyling, this subchapter is dedicated to you. In this chapter, we will explore the initial steps you can take to discover your talent and embark on a rewarding journey as a men's hairstylist.

Hairstyling is an art form that requires creativity, dedication, and a genuine passion for transforming hair into works of art. Whether you have always been fascinated by the power of a well-groomed beard or have recently developed an interest in men's hairstyling, this is the perfect place to start.

The first step in discovering your talent as a men's hairstylist is to educate yourself. Take the time to research different hairstyles, trends, and techniques. Watch tutorials, read books and magazines, and attend workshops or classes if possible. Building a strong foundation of knowledge will not only boost your confidence but also allow you to better understand the unique needs and desires of your potential beard clients.

Once you have gained a basic understanding, it's time to get hands-on experience. Practice on friends, family members, or even willing volunteers to refine your skills. Start with simple cuts and styles and gradually challenge yourself with more complex techniques. Don't be afraid to make mistakes – it's all part of the learning process.

Networking is another crucial step in your journey. Connect with established men's hairstylists, attend industry events, and join online communities to learn from experienced professionals. Surrounding yourself with like-minded individuals will not only provide valuable insights but also open doors to potential job opportunities or mentorship programs.

Lastly, embrace the power of experimentation. As you develop your style and technique, don't shy away from trying new things. Be bold, take risks, and push the boundaries of traditional men's hairstyling. Your unique approach will set you apart from the competition and attract a niche audience of beard enthusiasts who appreciate your creativity.

In conclusion, discovering your talent as a men's hairstylist requires dedication, education, practice, networking, and a willingness to experiment. By taking these first steps, you will embark on an exciting journey that will not only allow you to transform hair but also enhance the confidence and style of your potential beard clients. Get ready to unleash your creativity and become a master in the art of men's hairstyling!

Education and Training: From Novice to Professional

In the world of men's hairstyling, education and training play a pivotal role in transforming a novice hairstylist into a skilled professional. This subchapter delves into the importance of education and the journey from being a beginner to becoming a sought-after men's hairstylist.

Education is the foundation upon which every successful hairstylist builds their career. Aspiring hairstylists must undergo rigorous training in reputable institutions to learn the art and science of men's hairstyling. These institutions offer comprehensive courses, covering various aspects such as beard grooming, haircut techniques, product knowledge, and customer service.

During the initial stages of their training, novice hairstylists gain hands-on experience by practicing on mannequin heads and eventually real clients. This phase allows them to develop their technical skills, understand different hair types, and explore the latest trends in men's hairstyles. As they progress, they are exposed to more complex haircutting techniques, including fades, undercuts, and intricate beard grooming.

Beyond technical skills, education also emphasizes the importance of communication and interpersonal skills. A professional men's hairstylist not only excels in creating impeccable hairstyles but also establishes a strong rapport with their clients. They listen attentively, understand their client's style preferences, and offer expert advice to achieve the desired look. Education equips hairstylists with these crucial skills, ensuring a seamless and satisfying experience for potential beard clients.

Furthermore, education in men's hairstyling is a continual process. Hairstylists must stay updated with the latest trends, techniques, and products in the industry. Attending workshops, seminars, and industry events helps professionals refine their skills and expand their knowledge base. This ongoing education ensures that hairstylists can offer the most innovative and cutting-edge styles to their clients.

For potential beard clients, understanding the level of education and training a men's hairstylist possesses is essential. By choosing a hairstylist who has undergone thorough training, clients can trust that their beard will be in capable hands. They can expect a personalized experience, expert advice on beard grooming products, and a range of styling options that suit their unique facial features and preferences.

In conclusion, education and training are the stepping stones for aspiring men's hairstylists to transform into skilled professionals. The comprehensive courses, hands-on experience, and continuous learning help them master the art and science of men's hairstyling. For potential beard clients, choosing a hairstylist with a solid educational background ensures that their beard grooming needs will be met with expertise and precision.

Finding My Niche: The Appeal of Men's Hairstyling

As a potential beard client, you may think that finding the right men's hairstylist is a simple task. After all, how hard could it be to trim and shape a beard? However, there is much more to men's hairstyling than meets the eye. In this subchapter, we will explore the unique appeal of men's hairstyling and its importance in achieving the perfect beard.

Men's hairstyling is an art form that requires skill, creativity, and a deep understanding of facial features. A skilled men's hairstylist can transform a simple beard into a work of art, enhancing your overall appearance and boosting your confidence. But what sets men's hairstyling apart from other forms of hairstyling?

Firstly, men's hairstyling focuses on the specific needs and desires of men. Unlike traditional hairstyling, which often caters to women, men's hairstyling takes into account the unique characteristics of male hair and facial structures. A skilled men's hairstylist knows how to work with different hair types, from coarse and curly to fine and straight, ensuring that your beard looks its best.

Secondly, men's hairstyling embraces the ever-evolving trends and styles in the world of men's grooming. A professional men's hairstylist stays up to date with the latest trends, techniques, and products, allowing them to offer you a wide range of options to suit your personal style. Whether you're looking for a classic, clean-cut beard or a trendy and edgy design, a men's hairstylist can bring your vision to life.

Furthermore, men's hairstyling is not just about aesthetics; it's about creating a personalized experience for each client. A men's hairstylist understands that your beard is an extension of your personality, and they take the time to listen to your preferences and goals. They will collaborate with you to create a tailored grooming routine that suits your lifestyle and enhances your unique features.

In conclusion, men's hairstyling offers a specialized approach to beard grooming that goes beyond mere trimming and shaping. It combines artistry, technique, and a deep understanding of male hair and facial structures to create a look that is both stylish and authentic to who you are. By finding a skilled men's hairstylist who can cater to your unique needs and desires, you can unlock the true potential of your beard and elevate your overall appearance.

Embracing the Beard: A New Avenue for Creativity

In recent years, the world of men's grooming has undergone a remarkable transformation. Gone are the days when a clean-shaven face was the only acceptable standard of masculinity. Today, beards have emerged as a powerful symbol of style, personality, and self-expression. As a potential beard client, you have the opportunity to embark on a new avenue for creativity that can truly elevate your look and make a bold statement about who you are.

Welcome to "Embracing the Beard: A New Avenue for Creativity," a subchapter of the book "Confessions of a Men's Hairstylist: Insider Tips for Beard Enthusiasts." Written by an experienced men's hairstylist, this chapter is dedicated to unveiling the endless possibilities and benefits that cultivating a well-groomed beard can bring.

For too long, men's grooming has been limited to haircuts and basic shaving routines. However, the rise of the beard trend has opened up a world of options for men seeking to express their individuality. Whether you desire a rugged, full beard or a perfectly sculpted goatee, there is a beard style out there that can enhance your features and complement your personal style.

This subchapter explores the art of beard grooming, delving into the various techniques, tools, and products that can help you achieve the desired look. Discover the secrets of shaping, trimming, and maintaining your beard, as well as the best practices for beard care and hygiene. From beard oils to specialized brushes, you will learn about the tools of the trade that every beard enthusiast should have in their arsenal.

But embracing the beard is not just about aesthetics; it is also about self-discovery and confidence. When you choose to embrace

your facial hair, you are making a statement
about your identity and embracing a form of
self-expression. A well-groomed beard can
boost your self-esteem, exude masculinity,
and even become a conversation starter.

As a potential beard client, you have the
opportunity to work with a skilled men's
hairstylist who understands the intricacies of
beard grooming. They can guide you through
the process, taking into account your facial
structure, hair type, and personal style to
create a bespoke look that suits you perfectly.
With their expertise, you can transform your
beard into a work of art that reflects your
unique personality.

So, if you're ready to embark on a journey of
self-expression and creativity, "Embracing
the Beard: A New Avenue for Creativity" is
your guide to unlocking the potential of your
facial hair. By embracing your beard, you are
embracing a new chapter in your grooming

routine, allowing your creativity to shine and truly owning your style.

Chapter 2: Understanding the Art of Men's Hairstyling

The Importance of a Good Haircut: Enhancing Facial Features

When it comes to grooming, many men tend to overlook the importance of a good haircut. However, a well-executed haircut can make a significant difference in enhancing your facial features and overall appearance. As a men's hairstylist, I have witnessed firsthand the transformative power of a great haircut on my clients. In this subchapter, we will explore the reasons why a good haircut is essential for enhancing your facial features and why you should pay attention to your grooming routine.

First and foremost, a good haircut can frame your face and highlight your best features. Your face shape plays a crucial role in determining the most flattering haircut for you. Whether you have a square, round, oval, or triangular face, a skilled hairstylist can create a cut that complements your unique facial structure. By choosing the right haircut, you can draw attention to your strong jawline, high cheekbones, or any other feature you wish to accentuate.

Furthermore, a good haircut can help balance out your facial proportions. If you have a long face, for example, a haircut that adds width and volume on the sides can create the illusion of a more balanced face shape. On the other hand, if you have a round face, a haircut with added height on top can elongate your face and create a more angular appearance. Understanding these principles and working with a knowledgeable men's hairstylist can help you achieve a more harmonious and proportioned look.

In addition to improving your facial features, a good haircut can also boost your confidence and self-esteem. When you feel great about how you look, it radiates in your interactions with others. A fresh haircut can make you feel more put-together, professional, and stylish. It can give you that extra pep in your step, making you feel ready to conquer any challenge that comes your way.

To ensure that you always maintain your desired look, regular visits to a skilled men's hairstylist are essential. They can provide guidance on the best haircut for your face shape, recommend suitable grooming products, and offer styling tips tailored to your individual needs. By investing in your hair and grooming routine, you are investing in yourself and your overall well-being.

In conclusion, a good haircut is not just about trimming your hair – it is about enhancing your facial features and boosting your confidence. By working with a skilled men's hairstylist and choosing the right haircut for your face shape, you can transform your appearance and leave a lasting impression. Remember, grooming is not just for women; it is equally important for men to prioritize their hair and grooming routine. So, embrace the power of a good haircut and unlock your full potential.

Identifying Face Shapes: Choosing the Right Style

Welcome to the subchapter on identifying face shapes and choosing the right style for your beard. As a men's hairstylist, I understand the importance of finding the perfect beard style that complements your face shape. By understanding your unique facial structure, you can enhance your features and create a truly remarkable look.

When it comes to identifying your face shape, there are generally six categories: oval, round, square, rectangular, diamond, and triangular. Each shape has its own distinct features and requires different grooming techniques to highlight your best attributes. Let's dive into each one to help you find the perfect beard style!

1. Oval Face Shape: Lucky you! The oval shape is considered the most versatile. You can experiment with various beard lengths and styles, from short stubble to a full beard. Just make sure to maintain balance and avoid overwhelming your face.

2. Round Face Shape: To add definition and length, opt for a beard that lengthens your face. Try a square-shaped beard or a goatee with some length. This will create the illusion of a more angular and elongated face.

3. Square Face Shape: Emphasize your strong jawline with a well-groomed beard. A short, neatly-trimmed beard

or a classic goatee can soften your features and add a touch of sophistication.

4. Rectangular Face Shape: If you have a longer face, consider a fuller beard style to balance out the proportions. A medium-length beard or a goatee with some length on the chin can help create a more oval appearance.

5. Diamond Face Shape: With a narrower chin and wider cheekbones, you can rock a variety of beard styles. A short, well-defined beard or a chinstrap can highlight your unique facial structure.

6. Triangular Face Shape: To add width to your jawline, try a beard that is fuller on the sides and shorter on the chin. This will create a more balanced

look and draw attention away from a prominent chin.

Remember, these are general guidelines, and it's essential to consult with a professional men's hairstylist to find the perfect beard style for you. They can assess your unique facial features and provide personalized recommendations.

In conclusion, identifying your face shape is the first step in choosing the right beard style. By understanding your facial structure and working with a skilled men's hairstylist, you can achieve a beard that enhances your appearance and boosts your confidence. So, go ahead and embrace the power of a well-groomed beard that perfectly suits your face shape!

Tools of the Trade: Essential Equipment for Styling

As a men's hairstylist, having the right tools is essential to achieving the perfect beard style. Whether you're a potential beard client looking to maintain your facial hair or a stylist searching for the best equipment, this subchapter will guide you through the essential tools of the trade.

1. Beard Trimmer: A high-quality beard trimmer is the foundation of any beard styling routine. Look for trimmers with adjustable settings, different blade lengths, and a rechargeable battery for convenience. This versatile tool allows you to shape and maintain your beard with precision.

2. Beard Comb: A beard comb is a must-have for untangling and grooming your facial hair. Opt for a wide-toothed comb made of natural materials like wood or horn. It helps distribute beard oil, train the hairs, and ensure a neat appearance.

3. **Beard Brush:** Similar to a comb, a beard brush helps detangle and shape your beard. Look for brushes with boar bristles as they are gentle on your skin and help distribute natural oils, promoting a healthy and lustrous beard.

4. **Beard Oil:** Essential for maintaining a healthy beard, beard oil hydrates both the facial hair and the skin underneath. It helps soften the beard, reduces itchiness, and promotes a healthy shine. Choose an oil with natural ingredients and a pleasant scent to enhance your grooming experience.

5. **Mustache Wax:** For those looking to add a touch of personality to their beard, mustache wax is a game-

changer. It helps shape and style the mustache, keeping it in place throughout the day. Look for waxes with a firm hold and natural ingredients for a polished look.

6. Precision Scissors: To trim stray hairs or achieve intricate detailing, precision scissors are indispensable. These small, sharp scissors allow you to precisely trim your beard without risking any mishaps. Invest in a quality pair to maintain control and achieve professional results.

7. Electric Razor: While not essential for every beard enthusiast, an electric razor can be handy for maintaining a clean-shaven look or tidying up the edges. Look for a razor with multiple attachments to adapt to different styles and hair lengths.

Having the right tools is crucial for any men's hairstylist or beard enthusiast. By investing in high-quality equipment, you can achieve the beard style you desire while ensuring a comfortable and enjoyable grooming experience. Remember, proper maintenance and regular grooming sessions will help you rock the perfect beard with confidence!

Techniques and Tips: Mastering the Craft

Welcome to the subchapter dedicated to mastering the craft of beard styling and grooming. In this section, we will delve into the essential techniques and tips that every potential beard client should know, as well as provide insider insights from a men's hairstylist. Whether you're a seasoned beard enthusiast or just starting to embrace your facial hair, these tried-and-true methods will help you achieve the perfect beard.

1. Understanding Your Beard: Before diving into any grooming routine, it's crucial to understand your beard's unique characteristics. Is it coarse or fine? Patchy or dense? Knowing your beard's texture and growth pattern will help you determine the best techniques and products to use.

2. Trimming and Shaping: A well-groomed beard requires regular trimming and shaping. Invest in high-quality beard trimmers or visit a professional men's hairstylist for precise and tailored cuts. Remember, less is often more when it comes to trimming. Start with a longer length and gradually trim until you achieve your desired shape.

3. Beard Care Routine: Proper beard care goes beyond trimming. Maintain a regular routine that includes washing,

conditioning, and moisturizing your beard. Use a beard-specific shampoo and conditioner to keep it clean, soft, and free from irritation. Additionally, apply a beard oil or balm to keep your facial hair hydrated and healthy.

4. Brushing and Combing: Brushing and combing your beard are essential steps to tame unruly hairs and evenly distribute products. Opt for a boar bristle brush or a wide-toothed comb to prevent hair breakage and promote healthy growth. Brush or comb your beard in the direction of hair growth to maintain a neat appearance.

5. Styling Products: Experiment with different styling products to achieve your desired look. Beard balms, waxes, and gels can help shape and control your beard while adding a touch of style. However, remember to use these

products sparingly to avoid a greasy or weighed-down appearance.

6. Maintenance and Touch-ups: Regular maintenance is key to keeping your beard looking its best. Schedule touch-up appointments with a professional men's hairstylist to maintain the shape and health of your beard. They can provide expert advice on styling techniques and recommend any necessary adjustments.

Remember, mastering the craft of beard styling takes patience and practice. Embrace your individuality and experiment with different techniques and products to find what works best for you. By following these tips and seeking guidance from a skilled men's hairstylist, you'll soon have a beard that garners envy and admiration from all. Happy bearding!

The Psychology of Hair: Boosting Confidence and Self-Esteem

As a potential beard client, it's essential to understand the profound impact that hair, particularly facial hair, can have on your confidence and self-esteem. This subchapter explores the psychology behind hair and how it can be a powerful tool for boosting your overall sense of self.

Hair has always been a symbol of identity and self-expression. It holds the power to shape our perception of ourselves and how others perceive us. A well-groomed beard not only enhances your physical appearance but also influences your emotional well-being.

When you invest time and effort into maintaining a beard, it sends a message to the world that you care about your appearance. This self-care translates into increased confidence, as you feel more put together and in control of your image. People around you pick up on this confidence, and it can positively impact your personal and professional relationships.

Beyond the external factors, growing and grooming a beard can be a deeply personal journey. It allows you to embrace your individuality and assert your own unique style. Whether you opt for a full, bushy beard or a neatly trimmed one, your facial hair becomes a canvas for self-expression. This act of personalization can boost your self-esteem, as you proudly display a part of yourself that is entirely your own.

Furthermore, the act of grooming itself can be therapeutic. Taking the time to care for your beard can be a meditative practice, allowing you to focus on yourself and your well-being. This self-care ritual can reduce stress and provide a sense of calm in an increasingly fast-paced world.

A skilled men's hairstylist understands the psychological impact of hair and will work with you to create a beard style that suits your unique features and personality. They can guide you through the grooming process, providing tips and tricks to maintain your beard's health and appearance.

In conclusion, the psychology of hair is a powerful force in boosting confidence and self-esteem. By embracing your beard and investing in its care, you have the opportunity to enhance your overall sense of self. So, why not embark on this journey of self-discovery and let your beard be a reflection of your true inner confidence?

Chapter 3: The Beauty of Beards: A Deeper Look

The Rise of Facial Hair: Historical and Cultural Significance

In "Confessions of a Men's Hairstylist: Insider Tips for Beard Enthusiasts," we delve into the fascinating world of facial hair and its historical and cultural significance. This chapter explores the rise of facial hair, tracing its roots back to ancient times and examining its evolution throughout history. As a potential beard client and a part of the men's hairstylist niche, understanding the historical and cultural context behind facial hair can provide valuable insights into why it has become such a powerful symbol of masculinity and personal expression.

From ancient civilizations to modern-day trends, facial hair has played a significant role in various cultures worldwide. In ancient Egypt, for example, pharaohs and high-ranking individuals adorned their beards with gold and precious jewels as a symbol of power and authority. In ancient Greece, a well-groomed beard was associated with wisdom and masculinity, while in Rome, beards were a mark of virility and social status.

Throughout the Middle Ages, beards were subject to religious and cultural norms. In some periods, religious leaders deemed beards as unclean and sinful, leading to their removal. However, during the Renaissance, beards experienced a resurgence, becoming a symbol of intellectualism and sophistication.

Moving into the 19th and 20th centuries, facial hair took on new meanings. During the Victorian era, beards were seen as a sign of masculinity and respectability, with men meticulously grooming their facial hair to conform to societal standards. However, with the advent of the Industrial Revolution, a clean-shaven look became associated with professionalism and hygiene.

Fast forward to the present day, and facial hair has made an undeniable comeback. From the rise of the hipster beard to the popularity of the well-trimmed stubble, men are once again embracing facial hair as a means of self-expression. Beards have become a form of personal style, allowing individuals to showcase their individuality, creativity, and masculinity.

Understanding the historical and cultural significance of facial hair can help you make informed decisions about your own grooming choices. Whether you're considering growing a beard or seeking expert advice on maintaining your facial hair, this subchapter provides valuable insights into the rich tapestry of facial hair culture. As a men's hairstylist, I am here to guide you on your beard journey and ensure that your facial hair reflects your unique personality and style.

Different Beard Styles: Exploring the Options

As a men's hairstylist, I have had the privilege of working with countless beard enthusiasts over the years. One thing I have come to realize is that a beard is more than just facial hair – it is a statement of style and personality. Choosing the right beard style can make all the difference, enhancing your features and exuding confidence. In this subchapter, we will explore the various beard styles available to you, helping you find the perfect match for your unique look.

1. The Classic Full Beard:

If you're looking for a timeless and rugged look, the classic full beard is an excellent choice. This style requires patience, as it takes time for the beard to grow to its full potential. However, the result is a thick, well-groomed beard that exudes masculinity.

2. The Stubble:

For those who prefer a more low-maintenance option, the stubble beard is an ideal choice. This style is achieved by keeping the beard slightly longer than a clean shave, resulting in a rugged, effortlessly cool

appearance. It works well for both formal
and casual occasions.

3. The Van Dyke:

If you want to make a bold statement, the
Van Dyke beard is the way to go. This style
combines a mustache with a goatee, creating a
unique and distinguished look. The Van Dyke
requires regular maintenance to keep the
lines sharp and the facial hair well-groomed.

4. The Circle Beard:

For a more refined and polished look, the
circle beard is an excellent option. This style
combines a mustache with a rounded beard
that frames the mouth. It is a versatile choice
that works well for both professional and
casual settings.

5. The Garibaldi:

The Garibaldi beard is perfect for those who want to make a statement. This style is characterized by a full, rounded beard that is slightly longer and more unkempt than the classic full beard. It exudes a sense of confidence and individuality.

Remember, choosing the right beard style is a personal decision that should align with your face shape, lifestyle, and personal preferences. Consulting with a men's hairstylist can provide invaluable guidance in finding the perfect beard style for you.

In "Confessions of a Men's Hairstylist: Insider Tips for Beard Enthusiasts," we delve deeper into each beard style, providing detailed instructions on how to achieve and maintain the desired look. Whether you're a seasoned beard enthusiast or considering growing one for the first time, this book will serve as your go-to guide, helping you navigate the world of facial hair with confidence and style.

Unlock the potential of your beard and discover a world of possibilities. Embrace your individuality and let your facial hair reflect your true self. With the right beard style, you can elevate your style and leave a lasting impression wherever you go.

Beard Grooming 101: Essential Maintenance and Care

Introduction:

Welcome to the world of beard grooming! Whether you're a seasoned beard enthusiast or just starting to grow out your facial hair, it's important to understand the essential maintenance and care required to keep your beard looking its best. In this subchapter, we will discuss the key aspects of beard grooming, providing you with insider tips from a men's hairstylist's perspective.

1. Understanding Your Beard:

Before diving into the maintenance routine, it's crucial to understand your beard's unique characteristics. Every beard is different, and factors like hair density, texture, and growth patterns play a significant role in determining your grooming approach. Consulting with a professional men's hairstylist can help you identify the best grooming techniques for your specific beard type.

2. Washing and Conditioning:

Just like the hair on your head, your beard needs regular washing and conditioning to stay clean, healthy, and manageable. Use a mild beard shampoo or cleanser to remove dirt, oil, and product buildup. Follow it up with a nourishing conditioner to soften the hair and promote a healthy appearance.

3. Trimming and Shaping:

Regular trimming and shaping are essential to maintain a well-groomed beard. Invest in a high-quality beard trimmer or scissors to keep the length in check and create clean lines. A men's hairstylist can guide you on the best techniques to achieve your desired beard shape, whether it's a classic full beard, a stylish goatee, or a trendy stubble.

4. Beard Oil and Balms:

To keep your beard soft, moisturized, and itch-free, incorporate beard oil and balms into your grooming routine. These products work wonders in hydrating the hair and underlying skin, preventing dryness and flakiness. Experiment with different scents and formulas to find the one that suits your preferences and skin type.

5. Brushing and Combing:

Regular brushing and combing help distribute natural oils, detangle knots, and maintain a neat appearance. Use a boar bristle brush or a wide-toothed comb to gently untangle your beard, starting from the roots and working your way down. This simple step will enhance your beard's texture and overall look.

Conclusion:

Proper beard grooming is a combination of regular maintenance, good hygiene, and the right products. By understanding your beard's unique characteristics and following the essential care tips outlined in this subchapter, you'll be well on your way to maintaining a healthy, stylish, and envy-worthy beard. Remember, a professional men's hairstylist can provide personalized advice and guidance, ensuring your beard looks its absolute best. So, embrace the art of beard grooming and enjoy the journey to a well-tamed and irresistible facial hair style!

Addressing Common Beard Concerns: Itchiness, Patchiness, and more

Introduction:

Welcome to the subchapter on addressing common beard concerns! In this section, we will discuss some of the most prevalent issues that men face when growing and maintaining their beards. As a men's hairstylist, I understand the importance of a well-groomed beard, and I am here to provide you with insider tips and valuable information to help overcome these common challenges. Whether you are a potential beard client or simply an enthusiast looking for expert advice, this subchapter is tailored to address your specific concerns.

1. Itchiness:

One of the most common complaints among beard growers is itchiness. This discomfort can be attributed to dry skin, ingrown hairs, or even improper grooming techniques. Fear not, for there are several remedies to alleviate this annoyance. From using moisturizers and beard oils to exfoliating regularly, we will explore various strategies to keep your beard itch-free and healthy.

2. Patchiness:

Many men struggle with patchy beards, where hair growth is uneven or sparse in certain areas. This can be frustrating, especially when striving for a full and luscious beard. In this section, we will dive into possible causes of patchiness and suggest solutions such as beard fillers, specialized grooming techniques, and even alternative styles that can help conceal any patchy spots.

3. Beard Maintenance:

Maintaining a well-groomed beard is essential for achieving the desired look. From trimming and shaping to cleaning and conditioning, proper maintenance is crucial. We will discuss the right tools to use, step-by-step grooming routines, and the importance of regular visits to a men's hairstylist to ensure your beard remains in top condition.

4. Styling Tips:

Once you have addressed the common concerns and achieved a healthy and well-maintained beard, it's time to explore various styling options. From classic designs to trendy styles, we will discuss how to accentuate your facial features and create a look that best suits your personality and lifestyle.

Conclusion:

In this subchapter, we have covered some of the most common concerns faced by men when it comes to growing and maintaining their beards. By following the tips and advice provided, you will be well-equipped to overcome itchiness, patchiness, and other challenges that may arise during your beard journey. Remember, a well-groomed beard not only enhances your appearance but also boosts your confidence. So, embrace your facial hair and let it become a defining feature of your personal style.

Styling Your Beard: Adding Flair with Products and Accessories

Welcome to the subchapter on "Styling Your Beard: Adding Flair with Products and Accessories" from the book "Confessions of a Men's Hairstylist: Insider Tips for Beard Enthusiasts." In this section, we will explore the various ways you can enhance your beard's appearance by using the right products and accessories.

As a potential beard client, you may already know that your beard is more than just facial hair; it's a statement of your style and personality. By incorporating the right products and accessories into your grooming routine, you can take your beard to the next level.

One essential product for styling your beard is beard oil. This multipurpose product not only moisturizes your facial hair but also nourishes the underlying skin. It helps to

prevent dryness, itchiness, and dreaded beard dandruff, ensuring your beard looks healthy and well-maintained.

Another must-have product is beard balm. This versatile product adds both texture and hold to your beard, allowing you to shape and style it according to your preference. Whether you desire a sleek and sophisticated look or a more rugged and untamed appearance, beard balm is your secret weapon.

To tame unruly hairs and achieve a polished look, beard combs and brushes are essential. These tools help distribute product evenly, detangle knots, and promote healthy hair growth. Additionally, they provide a relaxing and therapeutic experience, stimulating blood flow to the hair follicles.

For those seeking a touch of individuality, the world of beard accessories offers endless possibilities. From stylish beard beads to vibrant bandanas or even novelty mustache wax, these accessories allow you to express your unique personality through your facial hair. Experiment with different styles and colors to find what suits you best.

Remember, as a men's hairstylist, I believe that your beard should be an extension of your personality and style. By incorporating the right products and accessories into your grooming routine, you can add flair and make a statement with your beard. So go ahead, explore the world of beard products and accessories, and let your facial hair become a true reflection of your individuality.

In the next subchapter, we will delve into the art of beard shaping and trimming. Stay tuned to learn the techniques that will help you achieve a perfectly groomed and well-defined beard.

Chapter 4: Navigating the Men's Grooming Industry

Finding the Right Hairstylist: Tips for Choosing a Professional

When it comes to grooming your beard, finding the right hairstylist is crucial. A skilled and experienced men's hairstylist can make a world of difference in the way your beard looks and feels. But with so many options out there, how do you choose the perfect professional for your needs? Here are some tips to help you make the right choice and find a hairstylist who will take your beard to the next level.

1. Do your research: Start by asking for recommendations from friends, family, or colleagues who have amazing beards. They can provide you with valuable insights and help you find someone who specializes in men's grooming. Additionally, take advantage of online platforms and read reviews about hairstylists in your area. Look for

professionals who have a strong reputation and a portfolio of satisfied clients.

2. Check their expertise: Not all hairstylists are created equal, and not all of them specialize in men's grooming. Look for professionals who have specific experience and training in working with beards. A men's hairstylist who understands the intricacies of beard trimming, shaping, and styling will be better equipped to handle your unique needs.

3. Schedule a consultation: Before committing to a hairstylist, schedule a consultation to discuss your beard goals and expectations. This initial meeting will give you a chance to assess the stylist's professionalism, communication skills, and overall understanding of your needs. Pay

attention to how well they listen to you and whether they offer suggestions based on your preferences.

4. Assess their products and tools: A good hairstylist should have access to high-quality products and tools specifically designed for beard grooming. During the consultation, ask about the brands they use and their recommendations for maintaining a healthy and well-groomed beard. A professional who invests in top-notch products shows their dedication to providing you with the best results.

5. Consider their pricing and availability: While it's important to find a hairstylist who fits your budget, don't compromise on quality. Look for a professional who offers competitive pricing for their services without compromising on expertise. Additionally, consider their

availability and whether it aligns with your schedule.

Remember, finding the right hairstylist is a personal decision. Trust your instincts and choose someone who makes you feel comfortable and confident in their abilities. By following these tips, you'll be well on your way to finding a men's hairstylist who will transform your beard into a work of art.

The Consultation Process: Understanding Client Needs

When it comes to getting the perfect beard style, understanding your needs as a client is crucial. As a men's hairstylist, my goal is to provide you with the best grooming experience possible, tailored to your unique preferences and lifestyle. This subchapter will delve into the consultation process, shedding light on how we can work together to achieve the beard style of your dreams.

The consultation process Is the foundation of any successful hairstyling experience. It is during this initial meeting that we get to know each other, discuss your goals, and determine the best approach to achieving your desired beard style. This process is not only about understanding the physical aspects of your beard but also about understanding your personality, preferences, and lifestyle.

During the consultation, we will discuss the various factors that influence your beard style. This includes considering your facial structure, hair type, and the image you want to project. By understanding these elements, we can create a beard style that not only suits you but also enhances your overall appearance.

Additionally, the consultation process allows us to discuss the grooming routine and products that will work best for you. I will provide you with valuable tips and insights on how to maintain your beard and keep it looking its best between appointments. Whether you prefer a clean-cut corporate look or a rugged, untamed style, I will guide you on the products and techniques that will help you achieve your desired look.

Furthermore, the consultation process is an opportunity for you to express any concerns, questions, or doubts you may have. I encourage open communication, as it allows me to provide you with the best possible service. Your satisfaction and comfort are my top priorities, and by addressing any concerns upfront, we can ensure a smooth and enjoyable grooming experience.

In conclusion, the consultation process is a vital step in achieving the perfect beard style. By understanding your needs, preferences, and lifestyle, I can tailor my services to create a beard style that not only reflects your personality but also enhances your overall appearance. Through open communication and collaboration, we can work together to achieve the beard of your dreams. So, sit back, relax, and let's embark on this grooming journey together, ensuring that you leave my chair feeling confident and satisfied with your new beard style.

Building a Relationship: Trust and Communication

In the world of men's hairstyling, building a strong relationship with your hairstylist is vital. This subchapter focuses on two key elements that are crucial in cultivating this relationship: trust and communication. As a potential beard client, understanding the importance of trust and effective communication will greatly enhance your overall hairstyling experience.

Trust is the foundation upon which any successful relationship is built. When it comes to your beard, trust is especially critical. As a men's hairstylist, it is my responsibility to listen to your preferences and deliver results that align with your vision. By establishing trust, you can rest assured that your beard is in capable hands. Trust also allows you to communicate openly and honestly about your needs and concerns, making it easier for both parties to work together towards a common goal.

Effective communication goes hand in hand with trust. As a potential beard client, it is essential to clearly communicate your desired beard style, length, and maintenance preferences. A good hairstylist will actively listen to your needs, provide expert advice, and collaborate with you to achieve the best possible outcome. Remember, communication is a two-way street, and your hairstylist should also communicate their ideas, techniques, and any limitations they may encounter.

To establish trust and effective communication, it is crucial to choose the right men's hairstylist. Look for someone who has experience and a strong reputation in the industry. Read reviews, ask for recommendations, and even schedule a consultation before committing to a particular stylist. This initial meeting will allow you to gauge their expertise, communication skills, and overall compatibility. Remember, building a relationship with your hairstylist is a long-term commitment, so take the time to find the right fit.

Once you have found a hairstylist you trust, maintain open lines of communication. Regularly discuss your evolving beard goals, ask for advice on grooming products, and be receptive to their professional suggestions. Trust your hairstylist's expertise while also staying true to your personal preferences.

In conclusion, building a strong relationship with your men's hairstylist is based on trust and effective communication. By understanding the importance of these elements, you can ensure a positive and successful hairstyling experience. Choose a hairstylist you trust, communicate your needs clearly, and be open to their expertise. Remember, a great beard is the result of a collaborative effort between you and your hairstylist.

The Art of Collaboration: Bringing Ideas to Life

In the world of men's grooming, collaboration is an essential ingredient in transforming ideas into reality. As a potential beard client, you might be wondering how the art of collaboration plays a role in achieving the perfect beard style. In this subchapter, we will explore the importance of collaboration between men's hairstylists and their clients, and how it can bring your beard ideas to life.

When it comes to grooming, a men's hairstylist is more than just a pair of skilled hands. They are artists who understand the nuances of facial hair, trends, and individual preferences. The key to a successful collaboration lies in open communication and a shared vision. By actively participating in the creative process, you can ensure that your beard style reflects your personality and desired image.

During your consultation, the hairstylist will ask questions to understand your grooming routine, lifestyle, and personal style. This information will guide them in recommending the most suitable beard styles that complement your facial structure and enhance your features. Remember, a beard is not a one-size-fits-all approach, and the hairstylist's expertise will help you navigate through the vast array of options available.

Once you have discussed your preferences, the hairstylist will share their professional opinion, taking into consideration factors such as maintenance, grooming techniques, and the latest trends. This collaboration allows for a balance between your desires and their expertise, resulting in a well-informed decision that you will be happy with.

As the collaboration progresses, the hairstylist will bring your ideas to life by meticulously crafting your beard. Their skilled hands and attention to detail will ensure that every stroke of the razor or trim of the scissors is precise, creating a beard style that is unique to you.

Furthermore, this collaboration extends beyond the initial styling session. Your hairstylist will provide guidance on beard care, grooming products, and maintenance routines, ensuring that you can maintain your desired look at home. By working together, you can achieve a long-lasting and effortlessly stylish beard that turns heads wherever you go.

In conclusion, the art of collaboration between men's hairstylists and potential beard clients is an integral part of bringing ideas to life. By actively participating in the creative process and leveraging the hairstylist's expertise, you can achieve a beard style that reflects your personality and enhances your overall appearance. Embrace the art of collaboration and watch your beard transform into a masterpiece.

Beyond Hair: Additional Services and Expertise

When it comes to grooming, men often focus solely on their haircuts and neglect other essential aspects of their appearance. At our salon, we are dedicated to providing a comprehensive grooming experience that goes beyond just your hair. Our team of expert men's hairstylists understands the importance of a well-groomed beard and offers a range of additional services to enhance your overall look and style.

1. **Beard Trimming and Shaping:** Maintaining a well-groomed beard requires more than just letting it grow freely. Our skilled hairstylists specialize in beard trimming and shaping techniques that will help you achieve the perfect style that suits your face shape and personal preferences. Whether you prefer a neat and tidy beard or a rugged, masculine look, we have the expertise to make it a reality.

2. **Beard Maintenance and Care:** Just like the hair on your head, your beard needs regular care and attention to keep it healthy and looking its best. Our team of men's hairstylists can provide you with expert advice on beard care routines, recommend high-quality products specifically designed for beard maintenance, and offer personalized grooming tips to ensure your beard remains soft, manageable, and enviable.

3. Beard Coloring: If you're looking to add a touch of sophistication or experiment with a bolder look, our salon offers professional beard coloring services. Our experienced hairstylists can help you choose the perfect shade that complements your skin tone and hair color, ensuring a natural and flawless finish. Whether you want to cover up gray hairs or add a pop of color to your beard, our expertise in beard coloring will leave you feeling confident and stylish.

4. Beard Styling: Just as a great hairstyle can transform your overall appearance, a well-styled beard can elevate your style to new heights. Our men's hairstylists are skilled in various beard styling techniques, from creating intricate designs to sculpting a beard that perfectly complements your facial features. With our expertise, you can

achieve a beard that makes a statement
and sets you apart from the crowd.

At our salon, we understand that grooming is
not just about haircuts but a holistic
approach to your personal style. Our team of
men's hairstylists is dedicated to providing
you with the highest level of service and
expertise, ensuring that your beard is as well-
groomed and stylish as your hair. Visit us
today and discover the difference our
additional services can make in enhancing
your grooming routine.

Chapter 5: Insider Tips for Beard Enthusiasts

Daily Care Routine: Advice for Maintaining a Healthy Beard

As a men's hairstylist, I understand the
importance of a well-groomed and healthy
beard. A beard is not just a fashion
statement; it represents your style and
personality. To help you maintain a healthy

and enviable beard, I have put together some essential advice that should be a part of your daily care routine.

1. Start with a Clean Slate:

Before you begin any beard care routine, make sure your beard is clean. Use a beard-specific shampoo and conditioner to cleanse and soften your facial hair. This will remove any dirt, excess oil, and product buildup, leaving you with a fresh canvas to work on.

2. Moisturize, Moisturize, Moisturize:

Just like the hair on your head, your beard needs moisture to stay healthy and soft. Invest in a good beard oil or balm and apply it daily. This will hydrate your skin, prevent itchiness and dandruff, and promote healthy beard growth.

3. Comb and Brush Regularly:

Regular combing and brushing are crucial for maintaining a well-groomed beard. Use a quality beard comb or brush to detangle your facial hair, distribute natural oils, and style your beard. This will help you achieve a polished and neat appearance.

4. Trim and Shape:

Regular trimming and shaping are essential to keep your beard looking sharp and well-maintained. Invest in a quality beard trimmer and learn the art of shaping your beard to suit your face shape. If you're unsure, consult with a professional men's hairstylist for expert guidance.

5. Watch Your Diet:

Your beard's health is not just about external care; it also depends on your overall well-being. A balanced diet rich in vitamins and minerals is essential for healthy hair growth. Include foods high in proteins, healthy fats, and vitamins like Biotin, Vitamin E, and Zinc to nourish your beard from within.

6. Protect Your Beard:

Shield your beard from harsh environmental factors such as pollution, sun damage, and extreme weather conditions. Use a beard balm or wax with SPF protection when stepping out in the sun and cover your beard with a scarf or mask in extreme weather conditions.

By incorporating these simple yet effective tips into your daily care routine, you can achieve and maintain a healthy, well-groomed beard that will leave others in awe. Remember, a well-kept beard not only enhances your appearance but also boosts your confidence. So, embrace your facial hair and take pride in your beard journey.

Trimming and Shaping: DIY Techniques for Beard Maintenance

Welcome to the subchapter on "Trimming and Shaping: DIY Techniques for Beard Maintenance" from the book "Confessions of a Men's Hairstylist: Insider Tips for Beard Enthusiasts." In this section, we will delve into essential grooming techniques that every potential beard client should know. Whether you are a seasoned beard aficionado or new to the world of facial hair, these tips will help you maintain a well-groomed, stylish beard from the comfort of your own home.

As a men's hairstylist, I understand the importance of a well-maintained beard. It serves as a powerful expression of your style and personality. However, achieving the perfect look requires regular upkeep. By mastering the art of trimming and shaping, you can elevate your beard game to the next level.

To begin, invest in a high-quality beard trimmer and a pair of sharp, stainless steel scissors. These tools will be your trusted companions throughout your beard grooming journey. When starting out, remember to always start with a longer setting on your trimmer and gradually decrease the length until you achieve your desired look. It's better to trim conservatively at first, as you can always go shorter if needed.

When it comes to shaping your beard, it's crucial to have a clear vision in mind. Consider your face shape and personal style to determine the best shape for your beard. Popular styles include the classic full beard, the well-defined goatee, or the trendy stubble look.

For precise shaping, a beard comb and a small, handheld mirror will be your go-to tools. Use the comb to align the hairs and trim any stray ones that disrupt the desired shape. Regularly check your beard from different angles using the handheld mirror to ensure symmetry.

Maintenance is equally important. Regularly clean your beard with a gentle beard shampoo and conditioner to keep it soft, healthy, and manageable. Apply a few drops of beard oil to moisturize the skin beneath and prevent itchiness. Brush your beard using a boar bristle brush to evenly distribute the oil and maintain a neat appearance.

In conclusion, mastering the art of trimming and shaping your beard is essential for maintaining a well-groomed and stylish look. With the right tools, techniques, and a clear vision, you can easily achieve the desired beard style from the comfort of your own home. Remember to invest in quality products and practice regular maintenance for a truly exceptional beard.

Overcoming Beard Challenges: Taming Unruly Facial Hair

For all the beard enthusiasts out there, we know that growing and maintaining a beard is no easy feat. It requires dedication, patience, and a whole lot of love for your facial hair. However, we also understand that sometimes, your beloved beard can become unruly and present a whole new set of challenges. But fear not, as we are here to guide you through the journey of taming your unruly facial hair.

One of the most common challenges faced by men with beards is dealing with wild, untamed strands. These rebellious hairs can stick out in all directions, causing your beard to lose its shape and appear messy. The key to taming these unruly hairs lies in regular grooming and maintenance. Invest in a high-quality beard brush or comb to keep your beard in check. Brush or comb your beard daily, following the direction of growth to train the hairs to lay flat. This will help maintain a neat and tidy appearance.

Another challenge that many bearded men encounter is dry and itchy skin underneath the beard. This can be quite uncomfortable and discouraging. To combat this issue, it is important to keep your beard and the skin beneath it well moisturized. Using a beard oil or balm will not only hydrate the skin but also nourish the hair follicles, promoting healthier growth. Make sure to massage the oil or balm into your skin and beard thoroughly for maximum benefits.

Trimming and shaping your beard is another crucial aspect of maintaining a well-groomed look. Regular trims will help control the unruly growth and keep your beard in shape. Consider visiting a men's hairstylist who specializes in beard grooming. They have the expertise and knowledge to sculpt your beard according to your desired style and facial structure, resulting in a polished and refined appearance.

Lastly, patience is key when it comes to managing beard challenges. Every beard goes through an awkward growth phase, and it may take time to achieve the desired look. Embrace the journey and remember that with consistent care and grooming, you will overcome any beard challenge that comes your way.

In conclusion, taming unruly facial hair can be a daunting task, but it is not impossible. By following these tips and tricks, you can overcome the challenges and maintain a well-groomed and enviable beard. Remember, a well-kept beard not only enhances your appearance but also boosts your confidence. So, embrace your facial hair journey and enjoy the process of taming your unruly beard.

Styling and Experimentation: Creating Unique Beard Looks

Welcome to the exciting world of beard styling and experimentation! In this subchapter, we will dive into the art of creating unique and eye-catching beard looks that will make you stand out from the crowd. As a men's hairstylist, I have had the pleasure of working with countless beard enthusiasts like yourself, and I am thrilled to share my insider tips with you.

Beards have become more than just a fashion statement; they are an expression of individuality and personality. With the right techniques and a touch of creativity, your beard can become a canvas for endless possibilities. Whether you want to achieve a rugged, trimmed, or sophisticated look, there are various styling techniques that can help you achieve your desired result.

Experimentation is key when it comes to discovering your unique beard style. Start by determining the shape and length that suits your face shape and personal preferences. From there, you can explore different grooming tools such as scissors, trimmers, and razors to refine your look.

One popular technique is the fade effect, where the hair is gradually trimmed shorter towards the neckline, creating a seamless transition from the beard to the skin. This technique adds a touch of sophistication and can be achieved by a skilled men's hairstylist.

Another exciting trend is the use of beard oils and balms to add texture, shine, and control to your beard. Experiment with different scents and compositions to find the perfect product that suits your beard type and desired style.

For those who crave a more daring look, why not try some creative shaping? With the help of a professional men's hairstylist, you can explore geometric patterns, intricate designs, or even opt for a dyed beard to make a bold statement.

Remember, the key to successful beard styling is regular maintenance. Invest in high-quality grooming products and visit your trusted men's hairstylist regularly to keep your beard looking sharp and well-groomed.

In conclusion, styling and experimenting with your beard is a fun and creative journey that allows you to express your unique personality. By following these insider tips and working with a skilled men's hairstylist, you can create a beard look that turns heads and sets you apart from the crowd. Embrace your individuality, and let your beard be a reflection of your style and confidence.

Expert Recommendations: Tried and Tested
Products

As a leading men's hairstylist and a
passionate advocate for beard care, I have
had the privilege of working with numerous
clients who share the same enthusiasm for
maintaining a well-groomed and
distinguished beard. Over the years, I have
come across a wide range of products that
claim to transform your beard game.
However, not all of them live up to their
promises. In this subchapter, I will share with
you my expert recommendations for tried and
tested products that will help you achieve the
perfect beard you desire.

1. Beard Oil: A good quality beard oil is
   an absolute must-have for any bearded
   gentleman. It not only moisturizes and
   nourishes your beard, but it also
   prevents itchiness and dryness. Look
   for products with natural ingredients
   like argan oil, jojoba oil, and essential
   oils such as cedarwood or sandalwood.

2. **Beard Balm:** If you want to tame and style your beard, a beard balm is your go-to product. It provides a light hold and helps shape your beard while adding a healthy shine. Look for balms with shea butter, beeswax, and essential oils for optimal results.

3. **Beard Shampoo and Conditioner:** Just like the hair on your head, your beard also needs proper cleansing and conditioning. Invest in a good quality beard shampoo and conditioner that are specifically formulated for facial hair. These products will keep your beard clean, hydrated, and free from any debris or odors.

4. **Beard Brush and Comb:** To maintain a well-groomed beard, you need the right tools. A high-quality beard brush and

comb are essential for detangling, shaping, and distributing beard products evenly. Look for brushes with soft bristles and combs with wide and fine teeth for different styling needs.

5. Beard Trimmer: For those who prefer a well-trimmed beard, a reliable beard trimmer is a must. Look for one with adjustable settings and different length guards to achieve your desired beard length. Remember to trim your beard when it's dry for more accurate results.

By investing in these tried and tested products, you can elevate your beard grooming routine and achieve the envy-worthy beard you've always desired. Remember, consistency and patience are key when it comes to beard care. Experiment with different products, techniques, and styles until you find what works best for you. Your beard is a reflection of your personality and style, so take pride in maintaining it with these expert recommendations.

Whether you're a seasoned beardsman or a newcomer to the beard world, these products are essential to your grooming arsenal. Trust in the expertise of a men's hairstylist and indulge in the art of beard care to elevate your grooming routine to new heights.

Chapter 6: Beyond the Beard: Hair Trends and Styling for Men

The Evolution of Men's Hairstyles: From Classic to Contemporary

In this subchapter, we will delve into the fascinating journey of men's hairstyles, tracing their evolution from classic to contemporary trends. As a men's hairstylist, understanding the history and progression of these styles is crucial in helping potential beard clients achieve the look they desire.

Men's hairstyles have always been influenced by various factors, including cultural norms, societal trends, and personal expression. Throughout history, we have witnessed a plethora of iconic hairdos that have shaped the way men present themselves. From the clean-cut styles of the 1920s to the rebellious looks of the 1960s, the evolution of men's hairstyles reflects the ever-changing nature of fashion.

The classic era of men's hairstyle" was characterized by sophistication and elegance. The 1920s introduced the sleek and polished look, with side parts and slicked-back hair. This style exuded confidence and refinement, epitomized by iconic figures like Clark Gable and Cary Grant.

As we moved into the 1950s, a more rebellious and youthful aesthetic emerged. Inspired by the rock 'n' roll culture, men started sporting pompadours and quiffs, defying conventional norms. Elvis Presley became a style icon, showcasing the versatility and creativity of men's hairstyles during this era.

The 1970s witnessed a shift towards longer hair and more natural looks. The hippie movement and the rise of counterculture influenced men to embrace their natural texture and grow their hair out. This era celebrated freedom of expression, with afros and shaggy hair becoming popular choices.

In the 1990s, the grunge scene brought about a disheveled and rugged look. Men began to experiment with unkempt hair, incorporating elements of rebellion and nonchalance into their style. Icons like Kurt Cobain became influential in shaping this trend.

Today, contemporary men's hairstyles are a fusion of classic elements with modern twists. The emphasis is on individuality and self-expression. From the sleek and sophisticated undercut to the trendy and versatile fade, there is a wide range of options for men to choose from.

As a men's hairstylist, it is essential to stay updated with the latest trends and techniques. By understanding the evolution of men's hairstyles, you can guide potential beard clients towards the perfect haircut that aligns with their personality, lifestyle, and desired image.

In "Confessions of a Men's Hairstylist: Insider Tips for Beard Enthusiasts," we will explore the intricacies of each hairstyle, providing valuable insights and practical tips to help you achieve the look you desire. Whether you prefer a classic, retro-inspired style or a contemporary, edgy haircut, this book will serve as your ultimate guide to navigating the ever-evolving world of men's hairstyles.

Trendsetting Celebrities: Inspiration for Modern Haircuts

In the world of men's grooming, there is a constant search for inspiration and the desire to stay ahead of the curve. One surefire way to achieve this is by looking up to trendsetting celebrities who effortlessly set the bar high with their unique and stylish haircuts. In this subchapter, we will delve into some of these iconic figures who have left an indelible mark on the hairstyling industry and discuss how you can draw inspiration from them for your own modern haircut.

One such celebrity who has become synonymous with trendsetting hairstyles is the dashing David Beckham. Known for his chameleon-like ability to pull off a wide range of haircuts, Beckham has proven time and again that he is not afraid to experiment. From his signature pompadour to his buzz cut, he has showcased versatility and an unwavering confidence that can inspire any man looking to make a statement with his hair.

Another trendsetting icon is the suave and sophisticated George Clooney. With his salt-and-pepper hair, Clooney has redefined what it means to age gracefully. His classic and timeless hairstyles, such as the slicked-back look or the short textured cut, are perfect for men who want to exude confidence and elegance.

For those seeking a more edgy and adventurous style, Jared Leto is a celebrity who can provide a wealth of inspiration. With his long locks, ombre coloring, and unconventional haircuts, Leto showcases a fearless approach to hairstyling that is sure to turn heads. His hairstyles are perfect for men who want to express their individuality and stand out from the crowd.

In addition to these celebrities, there are many others who have left a lasting impact on the world of men's hairstyles. From Brad Pitt's textured crop to Ryan Gosling's classic side part, each of these trendsetters offers unique and inspiring haircuts that can be tailored to suit your personal style and preferences.

As a men's hairstylist, it is crucial to stay updated with the latest trends and draw inspiration from these trendsetting celebrities. By understanding their hairstyles and techniques, you can offer your clients a wide range of modern haircuts that are both stylish and tailored to their individual needs.

In conclusion, trendsetting celebrities serve as a constant source of inspiration for modern haircuts. Whether you prefer a classic, sophisticated look or an edgy and adventurous style, there is a celebrity out there who can provide the inspiration you need. By staying informed and drawing from their hairstyles, you can offer your clients the latest and most stylish haircuts, ensuring that they leave your chair feeling confident and trendsetting themselves.

Hair Care for Men: The Basics of Healthy Hair

Introduction:

In this subchapter, we will delve into the fundamentals of hair care for men, focusing on the essentials of maintaining healthy hair. As men's hairstylists, we understand the importance of a well-groomed appearance, and a healthy head of hair plays a significant role. Whether you're sporting a trendy beard or not, these tips will help you achieve and maintain luscious locks.

1. Shampooing and Conditioning:

Regular shampooing and conditioning are crucial for maintaining healthy hair. Use a quality shampoo that suits your hair type and scalp condition. Massage the shampoo gently into your scalp, focusing on cleansing the roots. Rinse thoroughly to remove any product residue. Follow up with a conditioner to nourish and hydrate your hair, leaving it soft and manageable.

2. Choosing the Right Products:

Investing in high-quality hair products designed specifically for men can work wonders for your hair. Look for products that promote hair health, such as those enriched with natural ingredients like argan oil, keratin, or vitamins. Avoid using harsh chemicals or excessive styling products, as they can damage your hair and scalp.

3. Regular Trims:

Regular haircuts are essential to maintain the health and shape of your hair. Visit your men's hairstylist every 4-6 weeks to prevent split ends and promote healthy hair growth. Discuss your desired style and ask for recommendations on the best cut for your face shape and hair texture.

4. Protecting Your Hair:

Just like your skin, your hair needs protection from external factors. Shield your hair from excessive sun exposure by wearing a hat, using a leave-in conditioner with UV protection, or opting for hairstyles that cover your scalp. Additionally, limit your use of heat styling tools like hairdryers, straighteners, and curling irons, as they can cause damage and dryness.

5. Healthy Lifestyle Habits:

Maintaining a healthy lifestyle also contributes to the overall health of your hair. Stay hydrated, eat a balanced diet rich in vitamins and minerals, and exercise regularly. These habits promote blood circulation, which is vital for healthy hair growth.

Conclusion:

Taking care of your hair is a crucial aspect of grooming for men, regardless of whether you have a beard or not. By implementing these basic hair care tips, you can ensure that your locks are healthy, strong, and always looking their best. Remember, consulting with a men's hairstylist can offer personalized advice tailored to your specific hair needs. Prioritize your hair care routine, and enjoy the confidence that comes with a well-maintained mane.

Exploring Different Hair Textures: Tips for Curly, Straight, and Wavy Hair

Understanding and embracing your hair texture is crucial to achieving your desired beard style. As a potential beard client, it's important to recognize that different hair textures require different approaches when it comes to grooming and styling. In this subchapter, we will explore the unique characteristics of curly, straight, and wavy hair, providing you with valuable tips and insights to help you make the most of your beard.

Curly Hair:

Curly hair can be a blessing and a challenge at the same time. The key to managing curly hair is moisture and proper hydration. Investing in a quality conditioner and leaving it on for a few minutes before rinsing can work wonders for taming frizz and defining your curls. Additionally, using a wide-toothed comb or your fingers to detangle your beard gently is recommended to avoid breakage. Embrace your curls by using a curl-enhancing product that suits your hair type and experiment with different beard styles that complement your natural curl pattern.

Straight Hair:

Straight hair tends to be more prone to oiliness and can appear flat if not properly cared for. Regular washing with a gentle shampoo will help keep your beard clean and fresh. As straight hair doesn't naturally have much volume, using a lightweight styling product, such as beard oil or a volumizing spray, can add texture and body to your beard. Consider opting for beard styles that add dimension and movement to your straight hair, such as a well-groomed stubble or a fade with a structured beard.

Wavy Hair:

Wavy hair combines some aspects of both curly and straight hair. It offers versatility and natural texture that can be accentuated with the right techniques. Use a moisturizing shampoo and conditioner to maintain the health of your waves and prevent frizz. Applying a styling cream or mousse to damp hair can help define your waves and keep them in place throughout the day. Wavy hair is well-suited for a range of beard styles, such as a medium-length beard with tapered edges or a textured beard with a disconnected undercut.

Remember, understanding your hair texture is the first step towards achieving a well-groomed beard. Experiment with different products, techniques, and beard styles to find what works best for you. Consulting with a professional men's hairstylist who specializes in beard grooming can also provide you with invaluable advice tailored to your specific hair type. Embrace your unique hair texture, and let your beard reflect your individuality and style.

Styling Tips and Tricks: Achieving the Perfect Look at Home

Welcome to the subchapter on "Styling Tips and Tricks: Achieving the Perfect Look at

Home" from the book "Confessions of a Men's Hairstylist: Insider Tips for Beard Enthusiasts." In this section, we will share valuable insights and techniques to help you maintain and style your beard effortlessly in the comfort of your own home. Whether you are a seasoned beard enthusiast or just starting your grooming journey, these tips and tricks will elevate your grooming game.

1. Invest in quality grooming tools: To achieve a perfect look, it's crucial to have the right tools. A high-quality beard trimmer, a fine-toothed comb, and a pair of sharp scissors are essential for maintaining your beard's shape and length.

2. Understand your face shape: Different face shapes require different beard styles to enhance your features. Determine your face shape – whether it's round, square, oval, or triangular – and choose a beard style that

complements it. Experiment with different lengths and shapes to find the perfect match for your face.

3. Regular maintenance is key: Just like your hair, your beard needs regular maintenance to look its best. Trim it at least once a week to keep it neat and tidy. Use your trimmer with different guard lengths for precision, and don't forget to clean up the neckline and cheek line for a polished appearance.

4. Master the art of beard grooming products: Beard grooming products such as beard oil, balm, and wax are essential for maintaining a healthy and stylish beard. Beard oil will keep your facial hair moisturized, while balm and wax help shape and tame unruly hairs. Experiment with different products to find the ones that work best for your beard type and style.

5. **Embrace your unique beard texture:**
    Every beard is unique, and your
    beard's texture plays a significant role
    in how it looks. Embrace your natural
    texture and work with it rather than
    against it. Whether your beard is curly,
    straight, or somewhere in between,
    there are various styling techniques to
    enhance its natural beauty.

Remember, achieving the perfect look at
home requires practice and patience. Don't
be afraid to experiment with different styles
and techniques. And if you need professional
advice or a fresh look, don't hesitate to reach
out to a trusted men's hairstylist who can
provide personalized grooming tips and
recommendations. With dedication and the
right tools, you'll be well on your way to
rocking a perfectly styled beard that reflects
your unique personality and style.

Chapter 7: The Men's Hairstyling Experience: From Salon to Success

Creating a Welcoming Environment: Atmosphere and Ambiance

In the world of men's hairstyling, finding the perfect hairstylist who understands the art of beard grooming is like discovering a hidden gem. As a potential beard client, you deserve nothing less than a welcoming environment where you can relax, feel at ease, and trust your hairstylist's expertise. This subchapter is dedicated to uncovering the secrets of creating an inviting atmosphere and ambiance that will enhance your overall experience.

First and foremost, a men's hairstylist who truly values their clients knows that the environment plays a crucial role in establishing a positive connection. From the moment you step into the salon, you should be greeted with warm smiles and a friendly atmosphere. A well-designed waiting area with comfortable seating, tasteful décor, and perhaps some soothing music will set the tone for a relaxing experience.

To further enhance the ambiance, attention should be given to lighting. Soft, warm lighting creates a cozy and intimate atmosphere, making you feel more at ease. Harsh fluorescent lights can be off-putting, so a skilled men's hairstylist will opt for softer lighting options that promote a sense of tranquility.

Another aspect that contributes to a welcoming environment is the overall cleanliness and organization of the salon. A tidy workspace not only reflects the professionalism of the hairstylist but also ensures that you can fully immerse yourself in the experience without any distractions. The scent of the salon should also be pleasant, whether it's achieved through scented candles, essential oils, or air fresheners that create a refreshing and inviting aroma.

As a potential beard client, you deserve undivided attention and personalized care. A skilled men's hairstylist understands the importance of making you feel valued and heard. They will take the time to listen to your grooming goals, provide expert advice, and tailor their services to suit your individual needs. This level of attentiveness will make you feel comfortable discussing your beard concerns and confident in the hairstylist's ability to deliver exceptional results.

Ultimately, creating a welcoming environment with the right atmosphere and ambiance is essential for a men's hairstylist who truly understands the needs of beard enthusiasts like yourself. By paying attention to the small details, from the moment you walk through the door until the completion of your grooming session, a skilled men's hairstylist will ensure that your experience is nothing short of exceptional.

Enhancing the Client Experience: Extra Touches and Services

As a potential beard client, you may already know that finding the right men's hairstylist who understands the intricacies of beard grooming is essential. But did you know that a truly exceptional hairstylist goes beyond just a great haircut or beard trim? In this subchapter, we explore the extra touches and services that can elevate your client experience to a whole new level.

1. Personalized Consultations: A skilled men's hairstylist understands that each beard is unique and requires individual attention. They will take the time to sit down with you and discuss your desired look, facial features, lifestyle, and even your grooming routine. This personalized consultation ensures that

you receive a tailored service that suits your specific needs and desires.

2. Beard Care Education: A reputable hairstylist not only transforms your beard but also educates you on proper beard care techniques. They will share insider tips and tricks to maintain a healthy and well-groomed beard between visits. From recommendations for quality beard oils, balms, and brushes to advice on trimming and styling, you will leave the salon armed with knowledge to keep your beard looking its best.

3. Relaxing Hot Towel Treatments: Picture this – as you sink into the barber's chair, a warm and aromatic towel is placed around your face, creating a soothing sensation. This extra touch not only helps to open up your pores but also relaxes your facial

muscles, making the grooming experience more enjoyable and rejuvenating.

4. Premium Product Offerings: A top-notch men's hairstylist understands the importance of using high-quality products during your grooming session. They will have an array of premium beard oils, balms, waxes, and styling products that are specifically formulated to nourish and style your beard effectively. These products will not only enhance your beard's appearance but also promote its overall health.

5. Additional Services: To truly enhance the client experience, some hairstylists go the extra mile by offering additional services. These may include traditional straight razor shaves, head massages, or even complimentary beverages to

make you feel pampered and relaxed throughout your visit.

In conclusion, when seeking a men's hairstylist for your beard grooming needs, remember that the best ones understand the importance of enhancing the client experience. From personalized consultations to educating you on proper beard care and offering extra touches like hot towel treatments and premium products, these professionals strive to provide you with a grooming experience that goes beyond your expectations. So, sit back, relax, and allow your hairstylist to transform your beard into a work of art while you enjoy the luxurious treatment that you deserve.

Building a Clientele: Word-of-Mouth and Marketing Strategies

As a potential beard client, you may find yourself overwhelmed with the plethora of options available when it comes to finding a men's hairstylist who can cater to your specific needs. This subchapter will shed light on the importance of word-of-mouth and effective marketing strategies in helping you make an informed decision and ultimately achieve the perfect beard style you desire.

Word-of-mouth is a powerful tool in the world of grooming, and it can significantly influence your choice of men's hairstylist. When someone recommends a stylist based on their exceptional skills, attention to detail, and ability to craft remarkable beard styles, it speaks volumes about their expertise. These personal recommendations hold a lot of weight, as they come from individuals who have experienced firsthand the magic of a talented men's hairstylist. So, don't hesitate to ask friends, family, or even strangers whose beard styles you admire for recommendations.

Additionally, online reviews and testimonials can be valuable resources when searching for a men's hairstylist. Check out social media platforms, online forums, and dedicated grooming websites for feedback from satisfied clients. By doing so, you can gain insights into the stylist's abilities, professionalism, and the quality of their beard styling creations.

Marketing strategies also play a crucial role in helping a men's hairstylist establish their reputation and attract potential clients like yourself. Look out for hairstylists who actively engage with their audience through social media platforms, where they showcase their beard styling techniques and share valuable grooming tips. This demonstrates their commitment to their craft and their willingness to connect with the grooming community.

Furthermore, consider attending grooming events, where you can meet men's hairstylists face-to-face and witness their skills firsthand. These events often feature beard styling competitions and demonstrations, allowing you to evaluate different stylists and find one that resonates with your personal style and preferences.

In conclusion, building a clientele is a vital aspect of a men's hairstylist's success. By relying on word-of-mouth recommendations, seeking out online reviews, and engaging with stylists through various marketing strategies, you can ensure that you find a talented and skilled professional who can transform your beard into a work of art. Remember, the key is to do your research, trust the experiences of others, and seek out stylists who are passionate about their craft.

Developing Professional Skills: Continuing Education and Growth

In the ever-evolving world of men's grooming, staying ahead of the curve is essential for any men's hairstylist. As a potential beard client, you may be wondering why it's crucial for your hairstylist to continuously develop their professional skills through continuing education and growth. In this subchapter, we will explore the importance of ongoing learning and how it directly benefits you, the client.

Firstly, let's acknowledge that the art of styling and maintaining beards is a specialized skill that requires expertise and precision. By investing in continuing education, your hairstylist ensures that they are up-to-date with the latest techniques, trends, and products specifically tailored for beard care. This means they can provide you with cutting-edge services, ensuring your beard looks and feels its absolute best.

Continuing education also allows hairstylists to expand their knowledge beyond the basics. They can delve deeper into specific areas such as beard grooming for different face shapes, understanding beard texture and growth patterns, and troubleshooting common beard-related issues. By developing a comprehensive understanding of these factors, your hairstylist can offer personalized advice and solutions, catering to your unique needs.

Moreover, continuous learning fosters professional growth and confidence. By attending workshops, seminars, and industry events, hairstylists engage with fellow professionals and learn from experienced mentors. This exposure not only helps them refine their skills but also builds a network of like-minded individuals who can provide ongoing support and inspiration. Ultimately, this growth translates into a more fulfilling client experience, as your hairstylist can confidently offer innovative suggestions and recommendations.

As a potential beard client, it's important to seek out hairstylists who prioritize continuing education. Look for professionals who actively participate in industry conferences, pursue advanced certifications, and constantly seek out new knowledge. This

commitment to ongoing learning
demonstrates their dedication to their craft
and ensures that they are equipped with the
expertise to meet your unique beard
grooming needs.

In conclusion, the world of men's hairstyling
is constantly evolving, and it is crucial for
professionals to develop their skills through
continuing education and growth. By staying
up-to-date with the latest techniques and
trends, hairstylists can provide you with
cutting-edge beard grooming services.
Moreover, ongoing learning fosters
professional growth and confidence, resulting
in a more personalized and fulfilling client
experience. So, when searching for a men's
hairstylist, choose someone who values
continuing education – because your beard
deserves nothing less than the best.

Fulfillment and Satisfaction: The Joys of
Being a Men's Hairstylist

Welcome to the subchapter that delves into the incredible joys and satisfaction that come with being a men's hairstylist. As potential beard clients, it's essential to understand the passion and dedication that drives men's hairstylists to create the perfect look for you. From crafting impeccable beard styles to ensuring your overall grooming experience is exceptional, let's explore the world of a men's hairstylist.

For many men's hairstylists, the fulfillment of their craft lies in the transformative power of a well-groomed beard. The moment a client sits in their chair, they embark on a journey together to discover the ideal style that enhances their features and boosts their confidence. With every stroke of the razor and precise trim, a men's hairstylist brings out the best version of their client, making them feel like a million bucks.

What sets men's hairstylists apart is their deep understanding of the unique needs and desires of their clients. They recognize that each individual has a distinct personality, and their beard style should reflect that. A skilled men's hairstylist takes the time to listen, interpret, and collaborate with their clients, ensuring that the end result exceeds expectations. They cherish the opportunity to bring their clients' visions to life and witness the joy and satisfaction that radiates from them.

Beyond the artistry of crafting impeccable beard styles, men's hairstylists find immense fulfillment in building lasting relationships with their clients. They become confidants, friends, and advisors, creating a safe and welcoming space where men can share their grooming concerns and seek expert advice. Men's hairstylists are passionate about educating their clients, sharing insider tips and tricks to maintain their beard's health and style long after they leave the salon.

The satisfaction of being a men's hairstylist extends beyond the transformational aspect. It lies in the joy of connecting with diverse individuals from all walks of life, understanding their stories, and being a part of their grooming journey. Men's hairstylists thrive in the dynamic environment of a barbershop, where camaraderie and laughter fill the air, creating a sense of community that transcends mere hairstyling.

In conclusion, becoming a men's hairstylist is not just a profession; it's a calling that brings immense fulfillment and satisfaction. The ability to transform a beard into a work of art, build lasting relationships, and be a part of your grooming journey is what drives men's hairstylists to excel in their craft. So, dear potential beard clients, rest assured that when you choose a men's hairstylist, you're not just getting a haircut or a trim – you're embarking on an unforgettable experience that will leave you looking and feeling your absolute best.

Conclusion: Embrace Your Inner Beard Enthusiast: Confidence Through Grooming

Congratulations! By picking up this book, you've taken the first step towards transforming your beard into a powerful symbol of confidence and self-expression. Throughout this journey, we have explored the world of beard grooming and discovered the secrets that will help you unleash your inner beard enthusiast. Now, it's time to embrace this newfound knowledge and confidently groom your way to success.

As a men's hairstylist, I understand the importance of a well-groomed beard. Not only does it enhance your appearance, but it also acts as a reflection of your personality and style. A properly maintained beard exudes confidence and draws attention from others. It is a statement that says, "I take pride in my appearance and care about how I present myself to the world."

In this book, we have discussed various aspects of beard grooming, including trimming, shaping, and maintaining your facial hair. We have explored different styles and trends that can help you find the perfect look that suits your face shape and personal preferences. We have also delved into the world of beard products, from oils and balms to brushes and combs, to ensure that your beard remains healthy, soft, and manageable.

But beyond the physical aspects, grooming your beard can have a profound impact on your self-confidence. When you take the time to care for your beard, you are making a conscious effort to invest in yourself. This act of self-care not only improves your physical appearance but also boosts your mental well-being. The confidence you gain from a well-groomed beard will radiate outwards, positively impacting various areas of your life, from personal relationships to professional endeavors.

Remember, embracing your inner beard enthusiast is not just about following grooming techniques; it is about embracing your individuality and finding your own unique style. Your beard is a canvas, and you are the artist. Experiment with different looks, take risks, and have fun with your grooming routine. Your beard has the power to transform not only your appearance but also your outlook on life.

So, potential beard clients, I encourage you to embrace your inner beard enthusiast and embark on this exciting grooming journey. With the knowledge and techniques shared in this book, you have the tools to transform your beard into a symbol of confidence and self-expression. Remember, your beard is an extension of your personality, and by grooming it with care, you are sending a powerful message to the world – that you are a man who values himself and takes pride in

his appearance. Let your beard be your
ultimate statement of confidence.

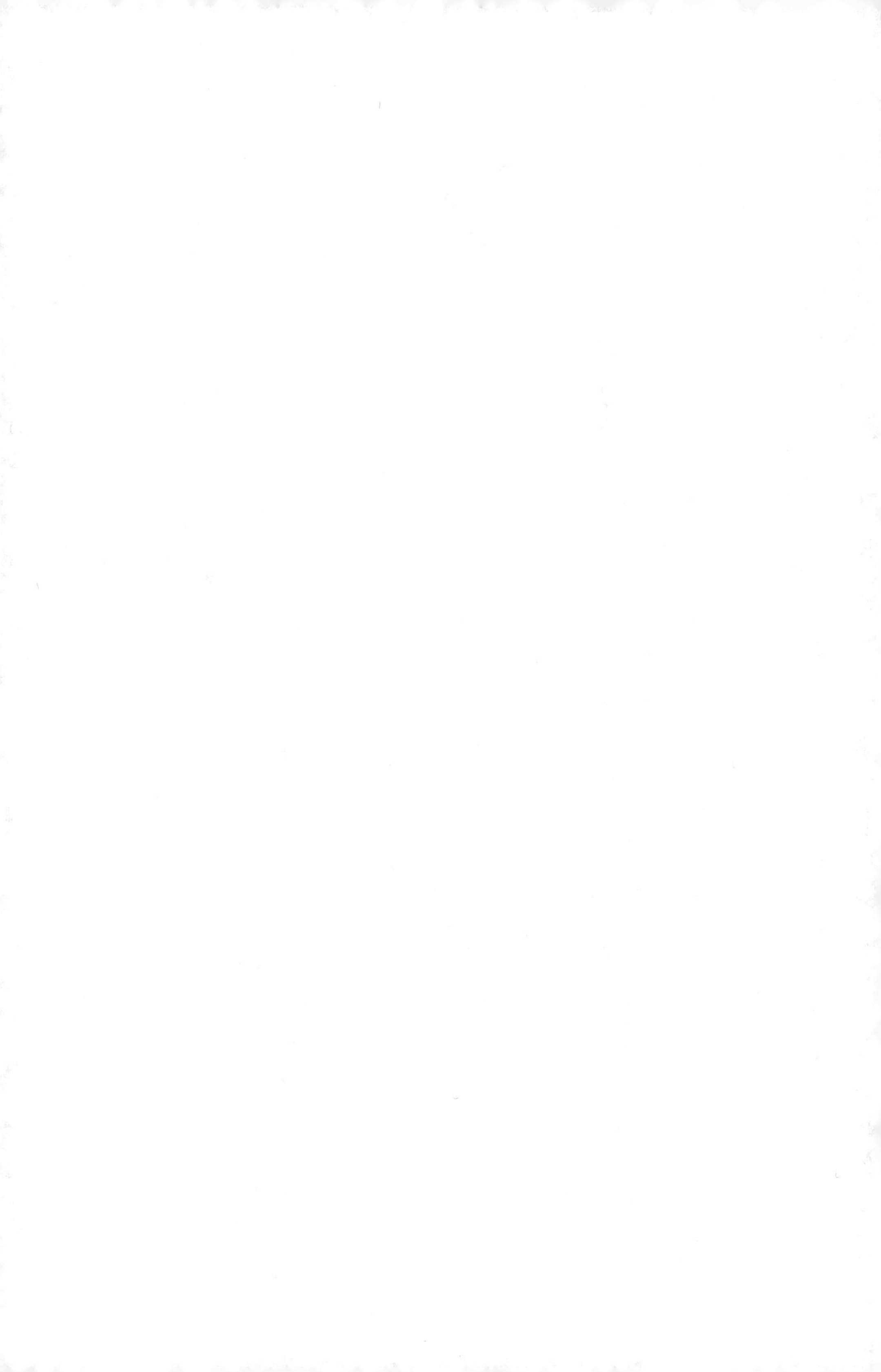

www.ingramcontent.com/pod-product-compliance
Lightning Source LLC
Chambersburg PA
CBHW050924260726
48660CB00001B/382